Wig Making Made Simple

By Master Wig Maker
Shon G. Stoker

Wig Making Made Simple

Copyright © 2012 by Shon G. Stoker

Every effort has been made to ensure that all the information in this book is accurate. However due to differing conditions, tools and individual skills, the author cannot be responsible for any injuries, losses, and any other damages which may result from the information from this book.

About The Author

Shon Stoker is a certified Paralegal, Hair Braider, Eyelash Extension specialist, Make Up Artist, Wig Maker, Entrepreneur and Author. However her most important roles are being a mother and a wife. She has worked in the modeling industry and has been featured in 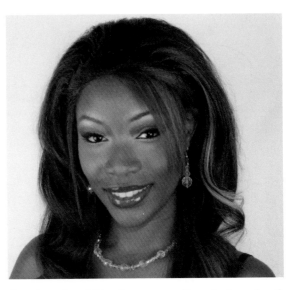 print ads, on the cover of national publications as well as being the face of Slim4us diet pill. After a few years in the modeling industry she decided to follow her passion in the beauty industry by creating her own wigs and hair pieces for models as well as using her natural talent as a professional makeup artist. After competing in a business plan competition Shon Stoker opened up her first shop in Houston, Texas. Shon is the owner of Enchanting Looks Houston formerly known as Lady S Hair Boutique. She now shares her knowledge with others and teaches the art of wig making.

For more info visit:
WigMakingMadeSimple.com

Table of Contents

Introduction to Wigs

Hair extensions cannot be worn by everyone, but anyone can wear a wig. Most of the flawless hairstyles celebrities wear are wigs. Now you can create the same wigs you see your favorite celebrity wearing.

After years of research I have created a way of learning wig making that makes creating your own wigs fun, understandable and simple with quality information a basic learner who wants to make wigs can use. With a few tools and supplies you can create beautiful, long lasting, custom wigs, using the information from this book.

Introduction Too Wigs

A woman's hair is her crown and a part of your overall appearance. A wig can help you look your very best. You can try a new look, hide thin or damaged hair, save time and money with an instant hairstyle.

The sales of wigs in the hair goods industry increased in the U.S and Canada from 200 million dollars to 900 million in the 90's to 2 billion in the 2000's according to Wigindustry.com. Wigs are the fastest growing products in the hair goods industry. Wigs are in demand and are here to stay.

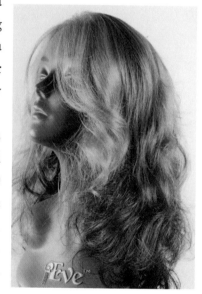

What is a Wig?

A wig is a head covering made of human or synthetic hair which covers the hair on the head, or a substitute for hair.

Wig Making is the art of adapting existing wigs or creating a wig from scratch.

Wigs have been around for thousands of years and a part of American culture for many years. Men and women have worn wigs since the earliest recorded time. Overtime wigs have ranged from elaborate styles to smaller hairpieces, toupees, wig lets, and braids. The overall purpose of a wig is to create your ideal look.

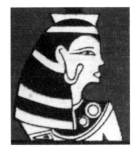

Types of Hair

Before beginning your first wig you must become familiar with the types of hair available for wig making. Educating yourself about the types of hair will give you an idea of what hair is best for the results of the wig you want to create.

Wigs became a major part of American fashion in the 60's and the demand for wigs soared. Wig manufacturers created synthetic hair just for the wig market. Synthetic hair is the most popular hair used in wig making.

What is Synthetic Hair?

Synthetic Hair - Man-made plastic fibers from Kanekalon, Toyokalon, or Monofiber that resemble human hair. Some synthetic hair is made with blended fiber and can sustain low heat. Synthetic hair usually melts when heat is applied. Most synthetic hair used in wig making comes with hair textures set in, and unlimited color availability from basic to fantasy colors.

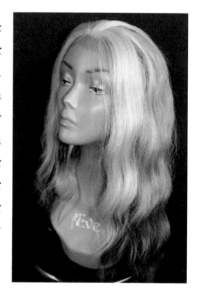

3 Most Common Types of Synthetic Hair

1. Kanekalon is a light, synthetic fiber that can withstand repeated washing and low temperature heat styling. It tangles and mats easily.

2. Toyokalon is a softer synthetic fiber that tangles less and is heat resistance, but lacks the natural look and color of Kanekalon fibers.

3. Monofiber is the highest quality synthetic hair. It has the realistic behavior, look and feel of human hair.

What is Human Hair?

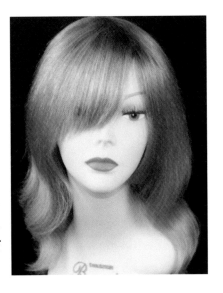

Human Hair is hair from the head of a human that goes through a stripping process of the cuticle known as an acid bath. This process places a silicone over the hair cuticle to give it shine and a smooth appearance. The hair can be colored, curled or permed.

Human Hair is classified by the donor's country of origin. Listed below are the most common types of human hair purchased.

The Five Most Common Types of Human Hair

1. Asian Hair is dense, thick, and straight, however it does not hold curls well.

2. Brazilian Hair is smooth with a lot of body and movement. The straight texture may wave up when wet.

3. European Hair is thinner, lighter with a silky feel that lays flatter than other types of human hair.

4. Indian Hair is one the most versatile. It holds lifts, curls, and adds color well.

5. Malaysian Hair has lots of body and waves up when wet.

Due to the way most human hair is processed, after a few washes and maintenance of the hair the silicone wears off and the hair loses its luster. You may want to consider a better quality of hair such as Remy or Virgin hair to lengthen the life of your wig.

Remy/Virgin Hair

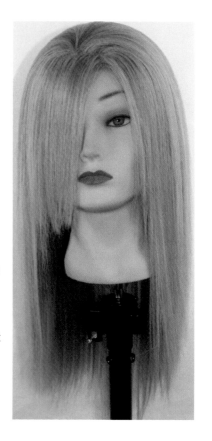

Remy and Virgin hair are processed differently from basic human hair. The process allows the hair to keep the look of luster longer. The donor's hair is cut close to the scalp in a ponytail. The hair cuticles, roots and follicles are kept in place and organized facing the same direction from root to tip. This allows for a reflective shiny appearance. The process ensures the hair remains soft, shiny, silky and tangle-free throughout its lifetime.

Remy Hair

Remy hair can be virgin, unprocessed, or processed. This means the hair can be colored, permed or relaxed, and the cuticle remains intact.

Virgin Hair

Virgin hair takes more time to harvest, because the hair is unprocessed. This contributes to the high premium price of this hair.

Virgin Remy hair last longer and is less likely to tangle than nonvirgin Remy hair. All virgin hair is Remy but not all Remy hair is virgin. Remy and Virgin hair are the highest quality of hair used in wig making. Top-quality Virgin European hair wigs are in high demand by those who desire to wear only the finest hair available.

Types of Wig Caps

Wigs come in a variety of cap constructions. The cap is the base of the wig that hair is attached to, using various techniques. Most wigs made are for the average person with a head size of 21 ½ to 23 ½.

Majority of wigs have the hair attached in "wefts" onto the cap. These are strings of hair doubled over and sewn closely together in long strands. The weft is then machine sewn or hand sewn to the wig cap.

The most common premade cap constructions are Standard wig cap, Monofilament wig cap, Dome cap, Nylon wig cap, and Lace front wig cap. The Standard, Monofilament and Lace front wig caps come with adjustable straps. You can also add your own straps, wig clips and combs.

Description of Wig Caps

1. Nylon Wig Cap is a cap made of nylon material. This cap is used to create wigs and aid the natural hair in laying flat under the wig. It offers elasticity to stretch the wig for a comfortable fit. Weft hair is glued or hand sewn to the cap.

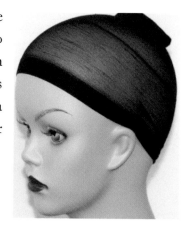

2. Standard Wig Cap is the most flexible and common of all the wig caps. It does not have an underlying solid cap, allowing the scalp to breathe. Wefts of hair are glued or hand sewn to the cap.

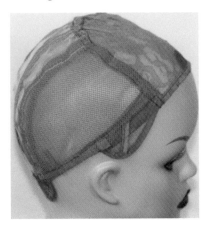

3. ¾ Cap has to be created using the standard wig cap by cutting or folding under and sewing down ½ to 1 ½ inches of the standard wig cap. You can sew or glue weft hair to the remainder of the base.

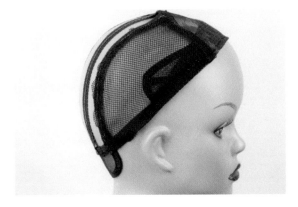

4. Dome Cap is a closed cap made of spandex material used to create a U-Shape wig. Weft hair can be glued or sewn to the cap.

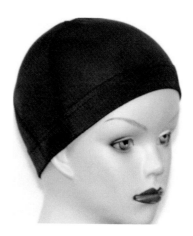

5. Lace Front Caps have the first ½ to 3 inches of the wig created of lace material with bulk hair ventilated to the lace and hair sewn or glued to the remainder of the cap.

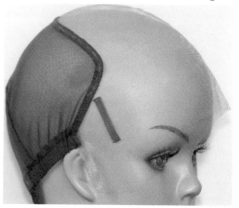

6. Monofilament Wig Cap is made of an elasticized mesh fiber. Hairs are ventilated at the front and crown where the mesh fiber is located. Hair can be glued or sewn to the remainder of the cap.

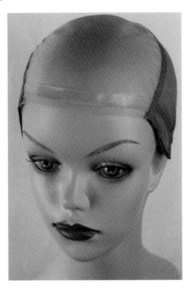

Wig Making Tools & Methods

After familiarizing yourself with the types of hair and wig making caps you must know wig making lingo. Learning the lingo will help you as you are creating your wigs you know what tools, techniques and supplies you are working with. (Reference Wig Glossary and Terms found in the back of the book.)

Wig Making Tool Kit

Ventilating Needles
Ventilating Needle Holders
Something to keep your ventilating needles in
Small Sharp Scissors
Seam Ripper
Slant Tipped Tweezers
Hand Sewing Needles
Curved Needles
Soft Tape Measure
Wig Caps (Standard Wig Cap, Nylon Wig Cap, Dome Cap, Monofilament Wig Cap, Lace Front Wig Cap)
Different colors of thread
Invisible Thread
Small Needle Nose Pliers
Haircutting Shears
Razor Blades
30 Second Bonding Glue
007 Bond Weave Crème
Blow-Dryer
Holding Spray

Wig Block, Wig Head or Mannequin Head
Wig Stand Tripod or Table Stand (To place wig head on)
Glue Gun
Cotton Jersey Headbands

<u>Wig Styling Tool Kit</u>

Rat Tail Comb
Wig Brush with wire bristles
Small & Wide Tooth Comb
Teasing Brush
Bobby Pins
Hairpins
Roller Pins
Wig T-pins
Duckbill clip
Wig Clips
Hot Rollers
Curling Iron
Flat-Irons
Rollers
Gel
Holding Spray
Spritz
Spray Mist Bottle

Wig Making Methods

Nylon Wig Cap

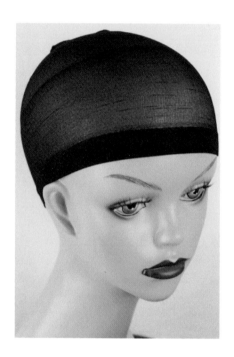

Tools Needed:
Nylon Wig Cap
30 Second Bonding Glue
Wig Brush
Blow-dryer
Small Scissors
Saran Wrap
Duckbill clip
Two bags of the weft hair of your choice (Synthetic or Human)

Holding Spray
Wide Tooth Comb
Rubber Bands
Wig Head
Wig stand

Step 1. Comb the natural hair straight back and braid the hair in a French braid. Place a rubber band at the end of the French Braid and tuck the braid under itself. Spray holding spray on any loose hair.

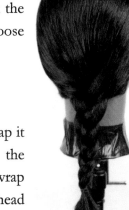

Step 2. Take the plastic saran wrap and wrap it around the head two times. After wrapping the saran wrap around the head twice, cut the saran wrap and fold the ends down.

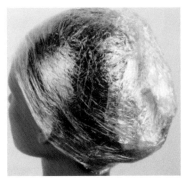

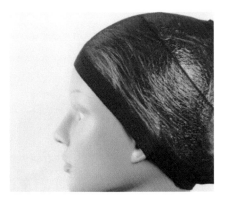

Step 3. Place the nylon wig cap over the head.

Step 4. Measure your first piece of weft hair from nape to nape and cut the weft hair. Place 30 Second Bonding Glue on the weft hair. Place the weft hair on the cap where you previously measured in the nape area. Do not to start at the bottom of the wig cap. (You can use holding spray on the cap and the weft to aid the bond to adhere to the cap. Use a blow dryer to assist the glue in drying faster.) Run your fingers across and press down to ensure proper bonding.

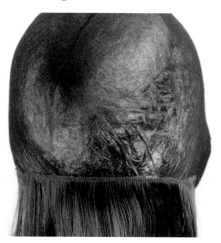

Step 5. Measure the next weft hair ½ inch or less above the last weft. Place 30 Second Bonding Glue on the weft. Put the weft hair on the cap. Repeat the process of measuring and gluing the weft hair from nape to nape and from ear to ear, then temple to temple creating a u shape.

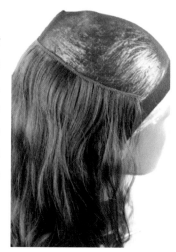

Step 6. The front and crown of the cap should not have any hair attached at this point. Measure the front weft between the two sides where you stopped the u-shape pattern. (Do not place wefts at the front edge of the cap.) Cut the weft hair and place the glue on the weft. You should have an oval shape in the middle of the head.

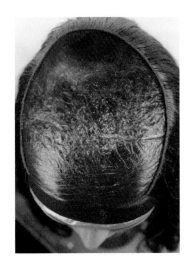 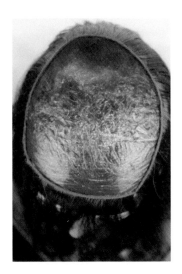

Step 7. Now you will close the top piece. Take a long piece of weft hair (about 1 ¼ feet long). Place glue on the weft hair, a few inches at a time. Glue the weft hair in a circular motion until you get a tiny circle in the top of the 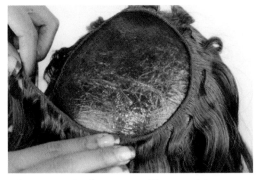 cap. (Leave a tiny hole open in the tiny circle, you will use this as an opening when closing the finished wig.) Make the circle as small as possible, leaving ½ inch of hair hanging.

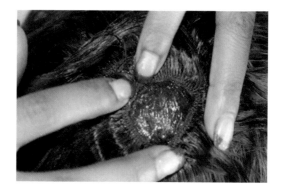

Step 8. Cut the weft hair that is hanging and place glue on the ½ inch of hanging hair. Allow the glue that you placed on the ½ inch weft hai to dry slightly.

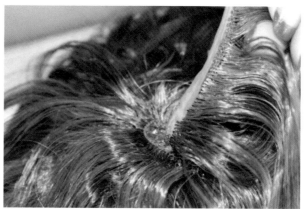

Step 9. Roll the hair in a circle going down.

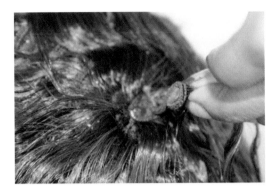

Step 10. Use the small circle of hair and tuck it in the small hole left open and spread the hair equally across for a natural falling of the hair.(You can use your curling iron or holding spray to make the hair lie flatter or tame any hair that is sticking out.

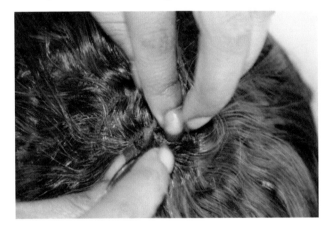

Step 11. Fill in spots where you would like to add more hair to make the wig appear thicker.

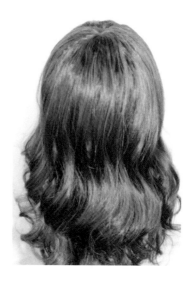

Now cut and style the wig to your desire.

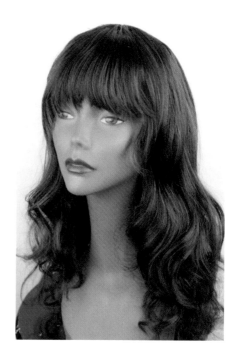

Standard Wig Cap

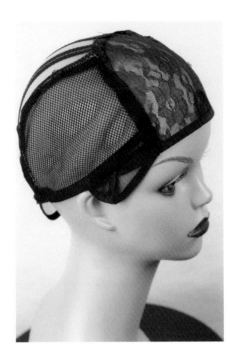

Tools Needed:
Standard Wig Cap
Thirty Second Bonding Glue
Curved Needle
Invisible Thread
Wig Brush
Blow-dryer
Small Scissors
Saran Wrap
Duckbill Clip
Two bags of the weft hair of your choice

Holding Spray

Step 1. Comb the natural hair straight back and braid the hair in a French braid. Tuck the braid under itself. Spray holding spray on any loose hair.

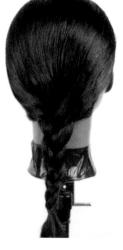

Step 2. Take the plastic saran wrap and wrap it around the head two times. After wrapping the saran wrap around the head twice cut the saran wrap and fold the ends down.

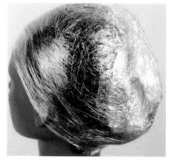

Step 3. Place the standard wig cap over the head.

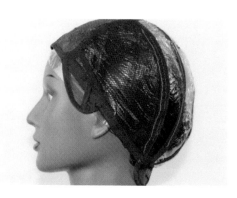

Step 4. Measure the first piece of weft hair from nape to nape and cut the weft hair. Place 30 Second Bonding Glue on the weft hair carefully. Put the weft hair on the cap where you previously measured in the nape area. Do not to start directly at the bottom of the wig cap. (You can use holding spray on the cap and the weft to aid the bond to adhere to the cap. Use a blow dryer to assist the glue in drying faster.) Run your fingers across and press down to ensure proper bonding.

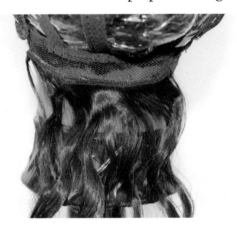

Step 5.   Measure the next weft hair ½ inch or less above the last weft hair. Repeat this process of measuring and gluing the weft hair from nape to nape and from ear to ear then temple to temple. (The back of this cap has areas where the cap is open. Place glue on the cap instead of the weft hair where the cap is open.) Place the weft hair on the cap slowly.

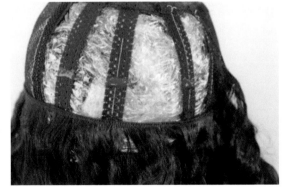

Step 6. The front and crown of the cap should not have any hair attached at this point. Measure the front weft between the two sides where you stopped the u-shape pattern. Do not place wefts at the front edge of the cap. Cut the weft hair and place the glue on the weft hair. You should have an oval shape in the middle of the head.

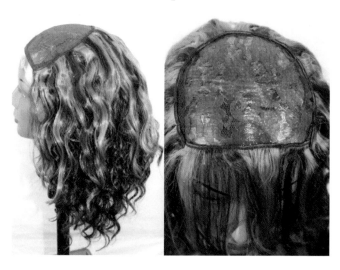

Step 7. Now you will close the top piece. Take a long piece of hair (about 1 foot long) place glue on the weft hair a few inches at a time. Glue the weft hair in a circular motion until you get a tiny circle in the top of the cap. (Leave a tiny hole open in the tiny circle, you will use this as an opening when closing the finished wig.) Make the circle as small as possible, leaving ½ inch of hair hanging.

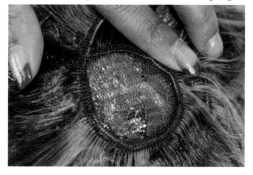

Step 8. Cut the weft hair that is hanging and place glue on the ½ inch of hanging hair. Allow the glue that you placed on the ½ inch weft hair to dry slightly.

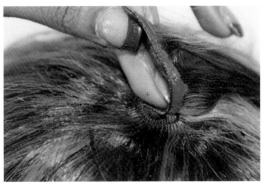

Step 9. Roll the hair in a circle going down.

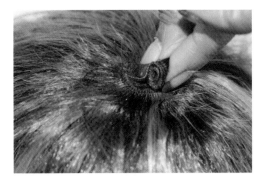

Step 10. Use the small circle of hair and tuck it in the small hole left open and spread the hair equally across for a natural falling of the hair.(You can use the curling iron or holding spray to make the hair lie

flatter or tame any hair that is sticking out.)

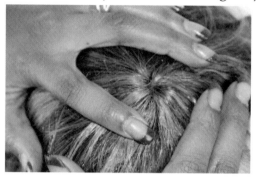

Step 11. Fill in spots where you would like to add more hair to make the wig appear thicker.

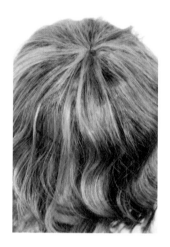

Step 12. Now cut and style the wig to your desire.

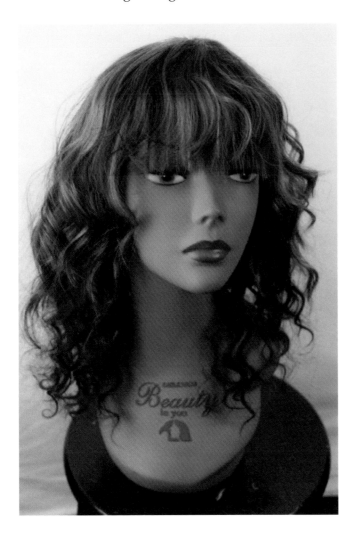

¾ **Wigs**

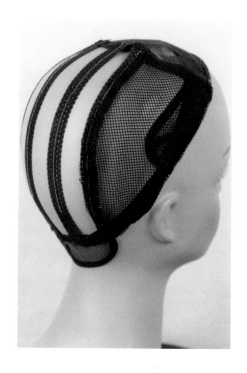

3/4 Wig Cap (Standard Wig Cap)

Tools Needed:
Standard Wig Cap
Thirty Second Bonding Glue
Curved Needle
Invisible thread
Wig Brush
Blow-dryer
Small Scissors
Saran Wrap

Duckbill clip
One bag of the weft hair of your choice
Holding Spray

Step 1. Fold the front 2 to 3 inches of the standard wig cap under and sew it down.

Step 2. Place the standard wig cap over the wig head.

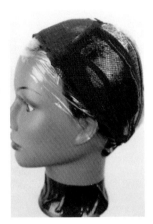

Step 3. Measure the first piece of weft hair from nape to nape and cut the weft hair. Be sure not to start directly at the bottom of the wig cap. Place the 30 Second Bonding Glue on the weft hair. Place the weft hair on the cap where you previously measured. (You can use holding spray on the cap and the weft to aid the bond to adhere to the cap. Use a blow dryer to assist the glue in drying faster.) Run your fingers across and press down to ensure proper bonding.

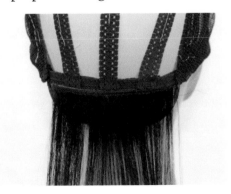

Step   4.   Continue measuring and bonding the weft hair to the pattern of the cap. (This cap has particular spots where the cap is open.) Place 30 Second Hair Bonding glues on the particular spots of the cap and attach the weft hair to the cap.

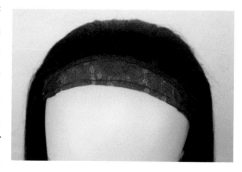

Step 5. Once the glue has dried, you can add wig combs to the front of the cap and wig clips in the back or the other way around. (You can also use bobby pins to pin the wig down to your head.)

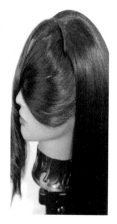

Step 6. Cut and style the wig.

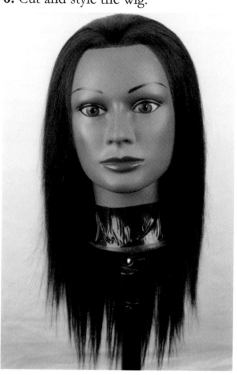

U-Shaped Wig

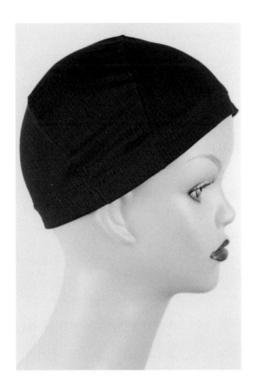

<u>Tools Needed:</u>
Dome Cap
Thirty second bonding glue
Curved Needle
Invisible thread
Wig Brush
Blow-dryer
Small Scissors
One bag of the weft hair of your choice

Holding Spray

Step 1. Comb the natural hair straight back in a French braid and tuck the braid under itself. Spray holding spray on any loose hair, so the hair lays flat. (I recommend creating this piece on a human head or a mannequin head with hair.)

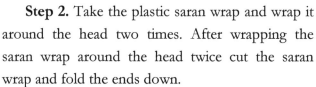

Step 2. Take the plastic saran wrap and wrap it around the head two times. After wrapping the saran wrap around the head twice cut the saran wrap and fold the ends down.

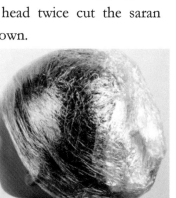

Step 3. Place the dome cap over the hair. Tuck all the hair into the cap. Allow the cap to stretch

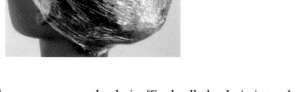

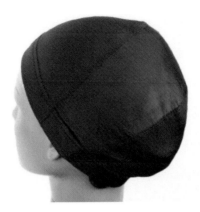

Step 4. Measure the first piece of hair from nape to nape. (Do not start at the bottom of the dome cap, because you will need this room to adjust and slide the wig on and off.) Place the 30 Second Hair Bonding Glue on the weft hair that you just measured. (You can use holding spray on the cap and the weft to aid the bond to adhere to the cap. Using a blow dryer can assist the glue in drying faster.) Run your fingers across and press down to ensure proper bonding.

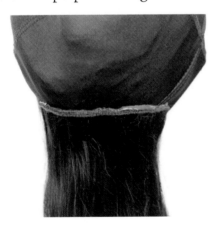

Step 5. Place the next weft hair ½ inch above the last weft hair in u-shape manner from ear to ear.

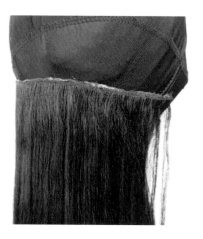

Step 6. Repeat this process until you cannot continue the u-shape pattern. The front edge of the cap and a small portion of the crown should be open. (The goal is to have the u-shape the exact size of the portion of hair you plan to pull out over the wig.) Do not place wefts a the edge of the cap.

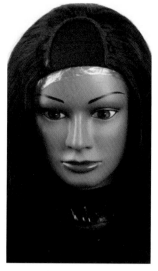

Step 7. Allow adhesive to dry. (You can sew the wefts down to ensure a secure bonding.) You should have a small u-shape in the front top of the cap. Cut the u-shaped area away.

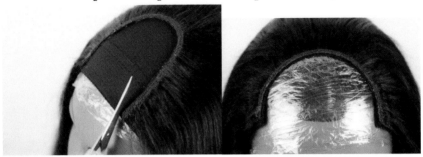

Step 8. Pull your hair out over the u-shaped area. You can add wig clips or use booby pins to attach the U-shaped wig.

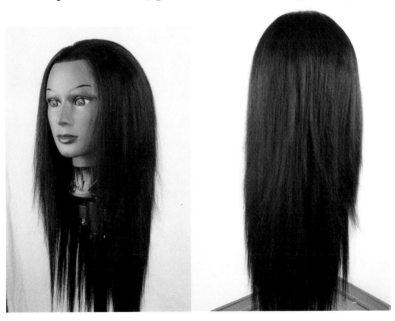

Lace Front Wig

(Requires ventilating hair)

Ventilating – The act of knotting hair to a wig lace to give the appearance that the hair is growing directly from the scalp.

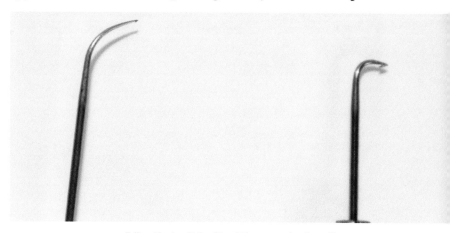

Ventilating Needles (German & Small)
(The German needle works best for ventilating monofilament and lace material. The small needle works best for lace material.)

Steps of How to Ventilate

Step 1. Hold the ventilating hook and holder in your dominant hand like you would hold a pen or pencil.

Step 2. Using a small section of bulk hair (ten to fifteen hairs in your left-hand if you're right-handed) fold it over. You should have a little less than two inches folded over. Pinch the loop of hair made tightly between the   thumb   and   index   finger   of   your   less   dominant   hand.

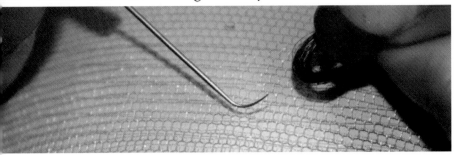

Step 3. Slide the ventilating hook under the hexagon hole or lace material that you have secured down to the wig block. Bring the loop of hair close enough to the hook to catch two to four hairs. (Don't bring the hook to the hair because this may cause your lace to stretch or tear.)

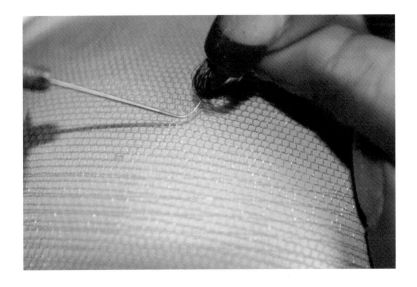

Step 4. After catching the hairs to the hook of the ventilating needle, pull the hair back under the lace material; turn the needle slightly to the left side. Be sure that you keep enough tension in the hand-holding the

hair and don't pull so far that the turned over end of the loop of hair pulls free.

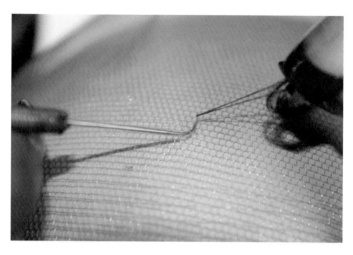

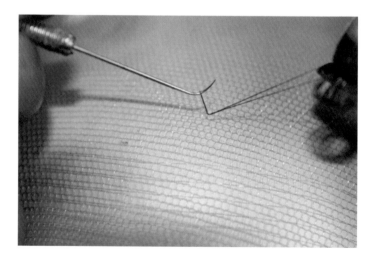

Step 5. Keep the loop of hair on the hook that you just pulled through the hole or lace material. Pull the hook, with the hair, back towards the hair in your hand. Wrap the hair in your hand over-the-top

of the needle and add a little tension when doing this. Turn the hook
away from you so it rests against the hair you just wrapped.

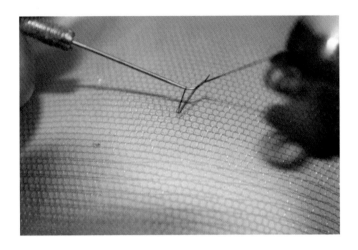

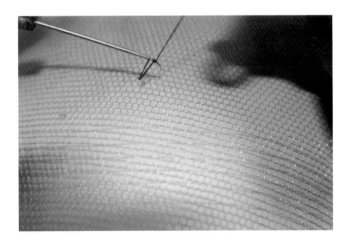

Step 6. Pull the hair you just wrapped around the needle through the
loop you made when you first started the knot. Pull the hair through the
loop and then tighten the knot. Continue ventilating the hair throughout
the lace.

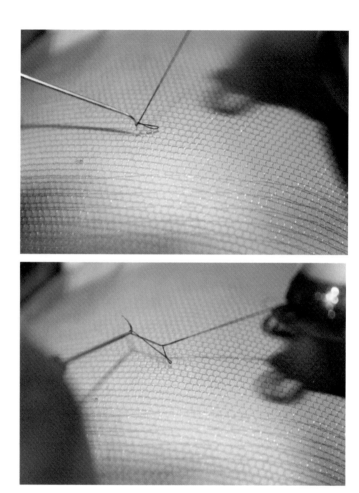

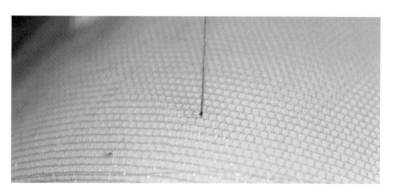

You can add baby fine, short or curled hairs and ventilate the hairs in the opposite direction of the wig around the perimeter to give the wig a more natural look.

Lace Front Wig

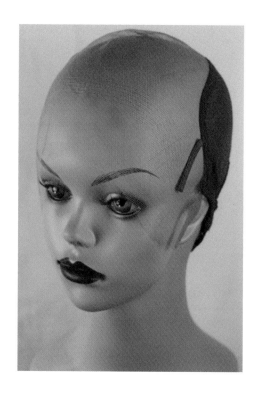

(Using a Premade Lace Front Cap)
<u>Tools Needed:</u>
Pre-Made Lace Wig Cap
Thirty second bonding glue
Curved Needle
Ventilating needle
Ventilating Needle Holder
Invisible thread
Wig Brush
Blow-dryer
Small Scissors

Duckbill clip
One bag of the bulk loose hair of your choice
One bag of weft
Holding Spray
Wig Block
Wig table head clamp or wig stand

Step 1. Place the premade lace front wig cap onto your mannequin head or wig block. You can Use T shaped wig pins to pin the lace front wig cap down or tape it down.

Step 2. Measure the first piece of weft hair from nape to nape. Do not start at the bottom of the wig cap, because you will need this room to adjust and slide the wig on and off. Place the 30 Second Bonding Glue on the weft hair carefully. (You can use holding spray on the cap and the weft to aid the bond to adhere to the cap. Use a blow dryer to assist the glue in drying faster.) Run your fingers across and press down to ensure proper bonding.

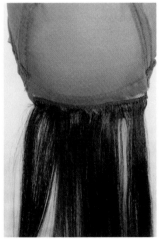

Step 3. Repeat the process of measuring and gluing the weft hair to the shape of the cap. (Once the hair wefts dry completely, you can sew over the tracks to ensure durable attachment.)

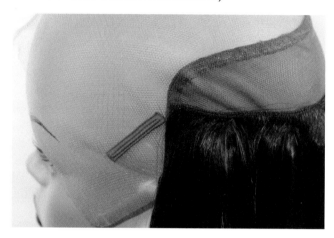

Step 4. Place your ventilating needle in the holder; you will begin ventilating the hair in the front part of the cap where the lace is attached (Refer to how to ventilate)The perimeter of the frontal will need to be ventilated one strand at a time for a more natural looking hairline. The remainder of the lace can be ventilated two to three strands at a time.

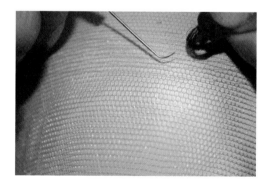

Step 5. Cut the excess lace from round the perimeter. Cut and style the wig.

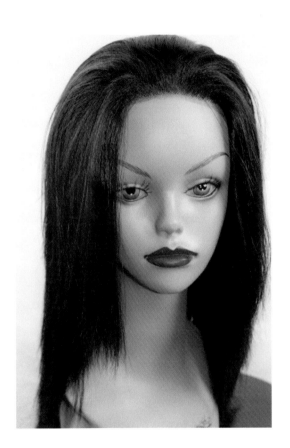

Monofilament Wig Cap

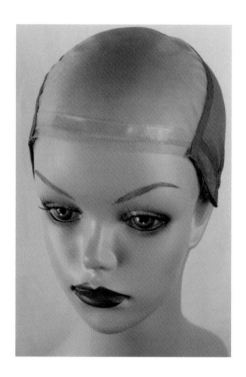

Tools Needed:
Pre-Made Monofilament Wig Cap
007 Bond Weave Crème
Curved Needle
Ventilating needle
Ventilating Needle Holder
Invisible thread
Wig Brush
Blow-dryer
Small Scissors
Duckbill clip

One bag of the bulk loose hair of your choice
One bag of weft hair
Holding Spray
Wig Block or Head
Wig Table Stand or Wig Stand Tripod

Step 1. Place the monofilament wig cap onto a wig block or mannequin head. Use T shaped wig pins to pin the monofilament wig cap down or tape the cap down.

Step 2. Measure the first piece of weft hair from nape to nape. Place 30 Second Bonding Glue on the weft hair. Do not to start at the bottom of the wig cap, because you will need this room to adjust and slide the wig on and off. (You can use holding spray on the cap and the weft to aid the bond to adhere to the cap. Use a blow dryer to assist the glue in drying faster.) Run your fingers across and press down to ensure proper bonding.

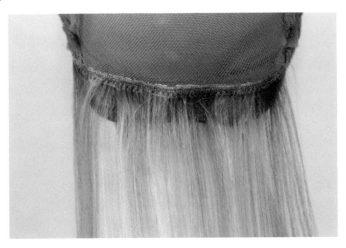

Step 3. Place the next weft hair about ½ inch or less above the las
weft hair from ear to ear. Repeat this step until you have a u-shap
pattern in the top of the cap. The front center and crown of the cap
should not have any hair attached at this point.

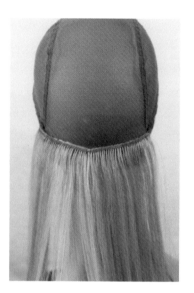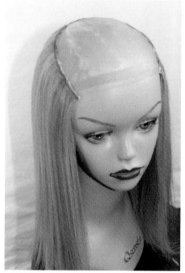

Step 4. Place your ventilating needle in the holder; you will begin
ventilating the hair in the front part of the cap where the monofilament
material is attached. The perimeter of the monofilament material will
need to be ventilated one strand at a time for a more natural looking hair

line. The rest of the
monofilament material
can be ventilated two
to four strands at a
time. (You can sew
over the tracks to
ensure   durable
attachment.)

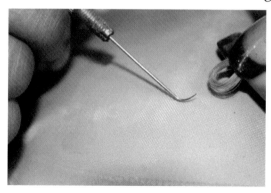

Step 5. Cut and style the wig.

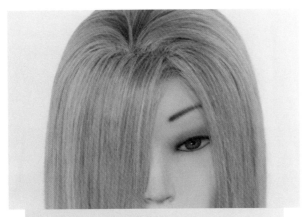

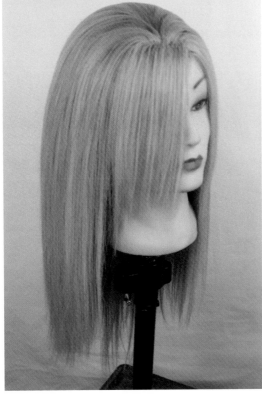

How to Make a Headband Wig

Tools Needed:
Hot glue gun
Glue sticks
Premade wig
Cotton jersey headband

Step 1. Place your premade wig on top of your wig head.

Step 2. Find the center part of the wig and the center of the underside of the jersey headband. Stretch the cotton jersey headband and place it over the wig.

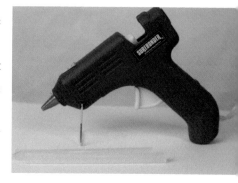

Step 3. Insert a hot glue stick into a hot glue gun, and let it heat for about 10 minutes. Place a generous amount of hot glue on the center of the wig with your glue gun and attach the cotton band. (Be sure stretch the band slightly.)

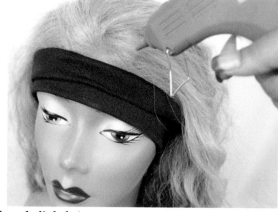

Step 4. Apply a thin line of hot glue horizontally around the perimeter of the wig and attach the headband pressing down firmly allowing the glue to spread evenly.

Step 5. Use a hair clip to hold the hair up in the back. Take the glue gun and place glue around the back perimeter of the wig from ear to ear. Attach the cotton band to the glue on the wig in the back and be sure to press firmly so the glue can spread evenly.

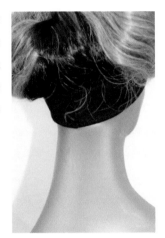

Step 6. Let the headband wig dry for 1-hour before wearing.

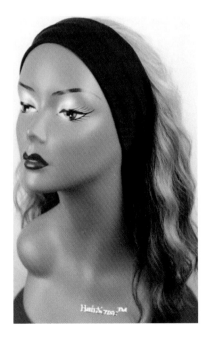

How to Make a Lace Front Headband

<u>Tools Needed:</u>
Premade Lace Wig
Sewing Needle
Clear thread
Cotton jersey headband

Step 1. Take premade lace front wig and cut the lace part of the wig. (This should be 1 ½ to 3 inches. Cut from ear to ear, cutting the lace from the rest of the wig.)

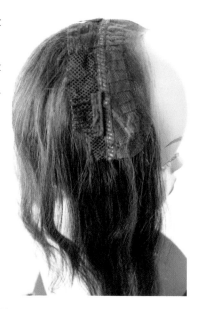

Step 2. After cutting the lace front, take the cotton jersey headband and cut 4 to 6 inches off.

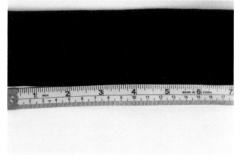

Step 3. Flip the lace front piece to the side with the lace. Take invisible thread and sew the end of the cotton jersey headband to the

ends of the lace front piece. Your results should be a lace front hairpiece with the cotton jersey headband attached to make a headband.

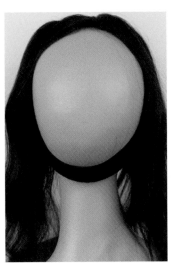

Step 4. Place the lace front headband over your hair and pull your hair through.

Step 5. Adjust and style your lace front headband.

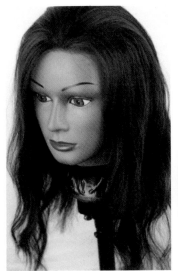

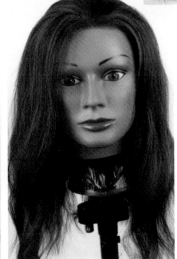

How to Attach the Different Wig Caps

There are different ways of attaching a wig. First decide whether the wig will be worn for a long period or short period of time. Then prepare the natural hair so the wig can be placed on top. Listed are a few suggestions on how to attach the different wig caps:

Standard, Nylon & Monofilament U-Shaped, ¾ Wigs are simple to attach. Secure the hair down using either braids or pin curls. You can place a nylon wig cap on top of your hair. You can also use bobby pins, add wig clips or combs to your wig.

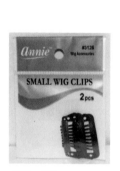
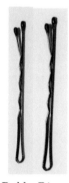
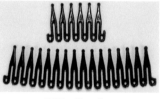

Wig Clips   *Bobby Pins*   *Wig Combs*

How to Sew Wig Clips into Your Wig

Tools Needed

Sewing Needle

Thread

Small Scissors

Wig Clips

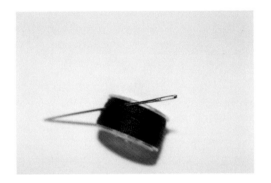

Step 1. Flip your wig inside out. Thread the sewing needle. Use a thread similar to the hair color of the wig to make the wig clips less noticeable.

Step 2. Take one of the wig clips and place the bottom of the clip at the bottom, middle portion of the wig. Make sure the teeth on the clip are facing you.

Step 3. Insert your sewing needle underneath the lace wig and then through the hole on the clip. Move to the next hole and insert the needle through the hole and then back down through the wig. Repeat this procedure until you have sewn through every hole on the wig clip.

Step 4. Place another wig clip about 3 inches away from the clip that you have just sewn onto the wig.

Step 5. Turn the wig to the right side about an inch above where your ear would be and sew another wig clip in this place. Repeat this same procedure for the left side of the wig. Don't attach any clips in the front of the wig, because it will be noticeable around your hairline.

Step 6. Flip the wig back into the right position and place it on you head. Insert the wig clips into your hair to secure the wig in place.

How to Glue Down Your Lace Front Wig

Tools Needed
Ultra Hold or Liquid Gold
Small Scissors
Rattail Comb
Wig Brush

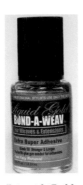 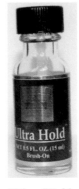

Liquid Gold   *Ultra Hold*

Lace Front Wigs- Liquid Gold and Ultra Hold are very popular adhesives if you choose to glue your lace front wig down. You can also attach your lace front wig using bobby pins, wig clips or sew your wig down.

Step 1. Cut away the lace border of your lace front wig.

Step 2. Set the lace front wig on your head and move it to your desired position. Line up the center part of the wig with the bridge of your nose and correct any placement issues.

Step 3. Once you have correctly placed the wig on your head. Fold the wig back so it will be out-of-the-way. Clean your forehead and hairline with alcohol.

Step 4. Apply the adhesive of your choice by using a small amount onto a small makeup brush or something like a nail polish brush and brush it along your hairline, creating a thin layer of glue.

Step 5. Allow the glue time to dry. (At least 15 minutes)

Step 6. Lay the lace border over the glue and gently press it down with your fingers this will seal the bond.

Step 7. After the lace border has been glued to your hairline, press your rat-tail comb handle down over the border. This will further secure the bond between the lace border and your skin.

How to Sew Your Lace Front Wig Down

Tools Needed

Curved Weaving Needle

Thread

Wig Brush

Scissors

Elastic Band

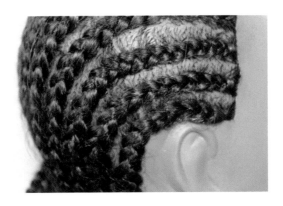

Step 1. Braid your hair in corn rows going straight back. (If you have long hair past the nape hairline, lift the braids upward and lay them between the corn rows and sew the braids together.

Step 2. Wipe your forehead at the hairline with rubbing alcohol to remove dirt and oil. This is where the lace will lie once the wig is on your head.

Step 3. Apply the scalp protector to the front hairline and let it dry.

Step 4. Place the wig on your head starting in the back and stretching it to the front. Align the frontal lace to your desired position.

Step 5. Place all of your wig hair up into a clip, leaving only an inch width of hair down around the back hairline and ears.

Step 6. Thread your needle.

Step 7. Sew the lace to the corn rows you created starting at one side of the head just above the ear and continue to sew moving along the back hairline until you reach just above the other ear. Use a slipknot to tie off the thread when complete.

How to Remove & Care for Your Wigs

A wig should be removed with the same care used to apply it.
Unpin or unglue the front. Most solvents will safely remove adhesive bonded lace wig. We recommend that you use the remover sold by the manufacturer and follow their directions.

If you used solvent give the solvent time to soften the glue and then carefully run the rounded end of a large wig pin under the lace to check that it is loose. Do not rush. Slip your hands up from the nape and carefully lift the wig up and slide it off the head. The wig should slide back off the head easily.

How to Clean & Care for Your Wig

Frequency of cleaning your wig will depend on your lifestyle and amount of perspiration. I suggest cleaning your wig after 7 to 12 days of wear.

Synthetic Wigs

Use shampoos, conditioners, hair sprays and other styling accessories designed specifically for synthetic wigs to care for synthetic wigs.

Human Hair Wigs

Human hair wigs are processed several times and it's vulnerable to damage. You can use any high quality shampoo formulated for processed hair. It is important to use hair care products which will help keep your wig supple, soft and healthy looking.

How to wash Synthetic & Human Hair Wigs

Step 1. Fill your sink with cool water. Add a capful of shampoo and blend in. If the wig has picked up the odor of smoke or other strong odors, you can add a teaspoon of baking soda to your water, and blend in.

Step 2. Gently, swish the wig in the water for about 30 seconds to a minute until the wig saturates completely with water.

Step 3. Gently scrub the front of the wig cap, where it meets the forehead until clean.

Step 4. Let the wig soak in the sink for about 15 minutes.

Step 5. Empty the sink of water and rinse the wig in cold water. It is important to use cool water on curly wigs; warm water will over-relax the curls of the wig.

Step 6. Gently squeeze excess water out of wig. Don't rub or twist your wig.

Step 7. Spread the wig out on a dry towel .Spray a little leave-in conditioner.

Step 8. Starting from the bottom, gently brush hair using a downward motion and gradually move up until all the hair is brushed. Do not begin brushing from the top or middle. The hair may tangle and become matted.

Step 9. Allow your wig to dry naturally overnight on a wig head.

When the wig is dry, restyle the wig gently shaking and fluffing your wig by hand is your best starting point for wig styling. Do not sleep in a wet or damp wig.

You can set your wig in rollers if desired.

Face Shapes

Identifying and understanding your face shape is the first step toward properly styling your wig. There is no right or wrong answer about your facial shape. When you have a good idea of your baseline shape it will help you select a flattering style for your wig.

How to identify your face shape:

To identify the shape of your face get a mirror and red lipstick. Look in the mirror and draw an outline of your face with your lipstick. You will be able to see the shape of your face. Compare it to the shapes and find the shape that is closest your facial structure.

Now you are ready to choose a hairstyle for your wig to compliment your good features and hide your flaws. Keep in mind the rule of classic proportions. The wig must not overwhelm you unless it is part of a theatrical look.

Here are seven of the most common facial structures and a quick style reference guide to help make sure your wig style for your wig suits you.

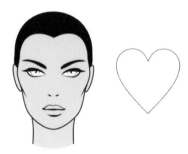

1. **Heart Shaped Facial Structure:** The forehead is the widest part of the face; it narrows gradually to the chin, which is slightly pointed.

Hair Part in your wig: Side parting is the best place to part your wig.

Recommended Styles: You want to decrease the appearance of your forehead width, while increasing the illusion of width on the lower part of the face. Chin length bob or long layers are great for your face shape. Up do hairstyles, with your hair 1/2 up 1/2 down with fullness focused on the down part adds balance to the face. Full curly bangs and wisps on your face look good on you. Adding curls and fullness to the chin area can also help round out the look of a heart shape face.

Styles to Avoid: Avoid pulling all your back into a slick style. Too much height and hair volume will lengthen your facial structure.

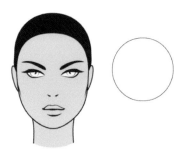

2. Round Facial Structure: Round at the cheeks with a circular forms, and heavier near the ears and gradually curves upward and downward.

Hair Part in your wig: Off center parts look great on your face shape.

Recommended Wig Styles – You want to create an illusion of length in the hair. Keep a focal point such as curls on top or tussled bangs to the side; this will draw attention away from the roundness of your face. Layered cuts with the height at the top but not at the sides compliment your features.

Styles to Avoid: Avoid slick back styles without hair touching your face and styles that are shorter than where your jawbone ends. Rounded styles will only make your face appear more round. Don't add width around the sides of your face, this will make the face appear to be wider than normal.

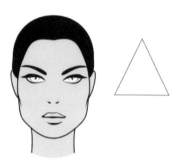

3. Triangular shape facial structure: This face shape has a wide chin and a narrow forehead.

Hair Part in your wig: Off center parts look best on this face.

Recommended Wig Styles: The main objective is to make your forehead look wider and your jaw smaller. Styles that give you more height on the crown area compliment your facial structure. Angle your wisps toward your face to soften the jaw line. Chin length, shags and wedge cuts that are full at the temples and taper at the jaw look the best.

Styles to Avoid: Long, full hairstyles that draw attention to jaw line and too much height at the crown.

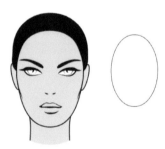

4. Oval shape facial structure: This facial shape is significantly longer than wide. The contour and proportions of the oval face form the basis for adapting all other facial types. Your facial features are well-balanced and almost every style will look great on an oval face.

Hair Part in your wig: Any part looks good on this face shape.

Recommended Wig Styles: Almost any hairstyle is possible for oval faces. Hair looks great pulled off your face. Bangs will accent your eyes and side swept bangs will cut across your forehead to soften it. Layers cut to an angle in toward your face will accent the feature where the angle ends.

Styles to Avoid: Wearing too much hair in your face because you want to show off those proportioned features.

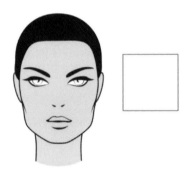

5. **Square shape facial structure:** Square jaw line, wide face, characterized by an angular jaw and square brow, with the jaw and brow being nearly the same width.

Hair part in your wig: Center part look best on this face.

Recommended Wig Styles: You want to balance the straight features of your face. Hair length is best about 1-1/2" below your chin. If you want to wear it up, add wisps around the face and bang areas. Curly up do's and messy side ponytail helps offset a strong jawline. Bangs and waves at the temple will soften the square shape facial structure. Rounded hairstyles will also break the square. Consider a body wave, or some curl to the hair.

Styles to Avoid: Long straight styles that accentuate square jawbone and straight flat bangs.

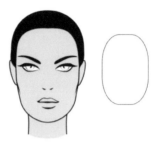

6. Oblong shape facial structure: Long, narrow shape, and or hollow cheeks.

Hair part in your wig: Side parting looks best on this face shape.

Recommended Wig Styles: Layers add softness to the straight lines in your face. Volume with an asymmetric flow of hair to one side widens and reduces length of your face. Straight falling bangs or bangs blended with the sides of your hair shorten the overall facial length. Curly and wavy styles add volume and width to your face. Up do's and slick back hairstyles look good on your face shape.

Styles to Avoid: Avoid any hairstyle that will lengthen your face.

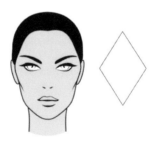

7. Diamond: Your facial features are wider cheek bones and a narrow jaw line and chin.

Hair part in your wig: Side parting is the best parting on this face.

Recommended Wig Styles: You want to wear styles that highlight the width of your face. Blunt cut bangs shortens the face length. Hairstyles that tuck the hair behind the ears are also complimentary for your facial structure. A chin length bob looks best because the haircut shows off your cheekbone structure.

Styles to Avoid: Styles with volume on top and styles without bangs.

Styling Tips

How to Create a Rooted Hairline

You can use any wig to create rooted hairline.

<u>Tools needed</u>
Duckbill Clips
Small Scissors
Rattail Comb
Teasing Brush
Holding Spray
Blow-Dryer

Step 1. Use your rattail comb, and part the hair about ¼ of an inch wide from ear to ear. Take the remaining hair and use a duckbill clip to clip the hair out of your way.

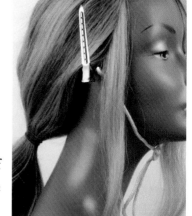

Step 2. Section off 1 ½ inches of hair, and clip the rest of the hair out the way.

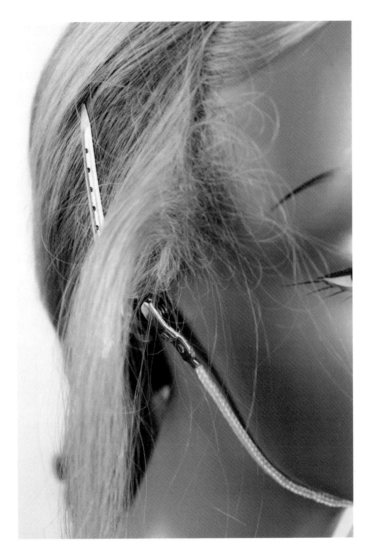

Step 3. Hold the hair up and back comb as close to the cap as possible and press down. Smooth the hair that was not back combed back to the rest of hair and clip it back.

Step 4. Repeat this process all the way around the wig front hairline.

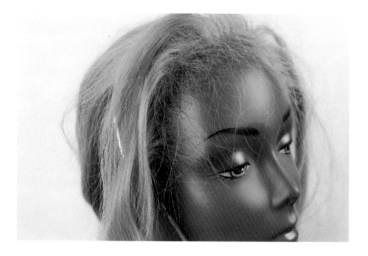

Step 5. Once the hair has been back combed and pressed down at the root. Use the holding spray and the tail of the comb, press down and blow-dry the hair. Be sure the backcombed hair is as flat as possible to the wig cap and the rest of the hair is combed out.

Step 6. Once the hair is rooted and sprayed remove the wig from the wig head and lay the wig on its back. Using the small scissors cut into the hair at an angle across the wig line.

Step 7. Spray the wig line with more holding spray and blow-dry.

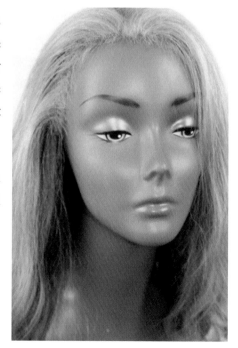

How to Create Bangs

Tools Needed

Small Scissors

Small Tooth Comb

Elastic Band

Duckbill Clips

Step 1. Part the hair where you want to create the bangs on your wig.

Step 2. Pull the remaining hair back out of the way. You can also use clips to clip the hair out of the way.

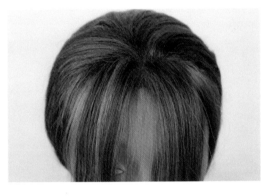

Step 3. Take your comb and slide the comb under the hair you left out to create the bangs. Make sure the teeth of the comb are facing outward.

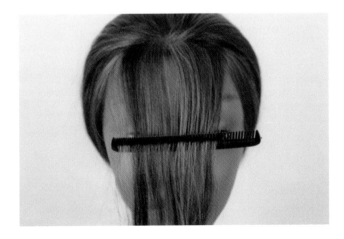

Step 4. Use a sharp pair of scissors (preferably scissors for haircutting) snip small bits at a time, tilting the scissors just a little bit at a downward angle. Do not cut straight across unless you want blunt cut bangs.

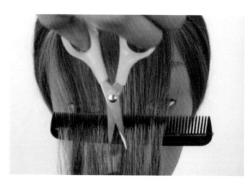

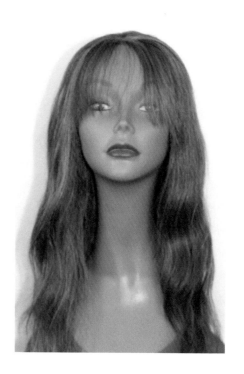

(After)Bangs

How to Create Curly Hair

Tools Needed
Curling Iron or Hot Rollers
Holding Spray
Comb
Wig Brush

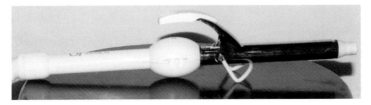

Curling Iron

If your wig hair is made of human hair you can use a curling iron or hot roller. (Some synthetic hair can sustain some low heat hot rollers.)

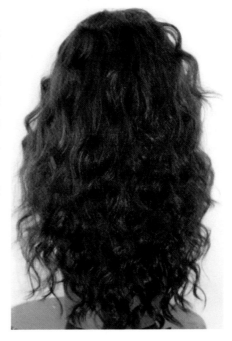

Step 1. Take the hair and part it in small sections and curl the hair using the iron. If you're using hot rollers section off the hair using your clips and roll the hair with the hot rollers and leave them in for no less than thirty minutes.

Step 2. Add holding spray for a maximum hold.

How to Create Pin Curls

Tools Needed

Comb

Wig Brush

Bobby Pins

Holding Spray

Step 1. Wet the wig hair and section out in 1-inch hair sections and roll them around with your index finger.

Step 2. Once secured, push the curl to the root of the head with your hand and place two bobby pins in the hair to hold the curl in place. The first bobby pin should go straight across the middle of the curl to anchor it to the hair and the second bobby pin should go in the hair at an angle perpendicular to the first bobby pin. The result should appear as if the bobby pins are making the letter "X" on top of the curl.

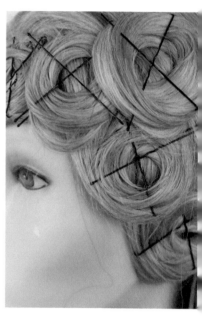

Step 3. Repeat the pinning process until the whole head is pin curled and leave the style to set for at least 8 hours. (I recommend leaving the wig overnight to dry so it may set properly.)

Step 4. After the required setting time remove the pins and gently shape the curls with your finger. Comb the hair as you like for a look simple yet elegant.

How to Create Straight Hair

Tools Needed

Flat Iron or Small Hand Held Steamer

Comb

Wig Brush

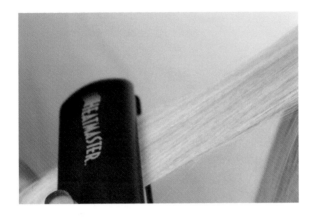

To create straight hair with your wig, use the straightening iron. Take the hair in small sections and straighten it with the flat iron, from root to end. If the hair is synthetic use a small hand held steamer. Comb and steam the hair from root to tip.

How to Create an Up Do

<u>Tools Needed</u>

Small Tooth Comb

Wide Tooth Comb

Wig Brush

Bobby Pins

Clear Rubber Bands

Chin Strap

Step 1. To create an up do with your wig make sure the sides of the wig are secured down on the head or wig block. Chin straps are useful when creating up dos.

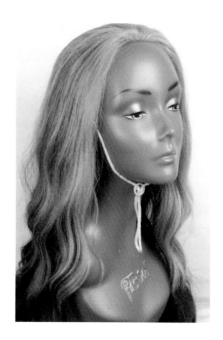

Step 2. Brush the hair up. Decide whether you want the hair in a bun, loose and curly at the nape of your neck, the middle or high up.

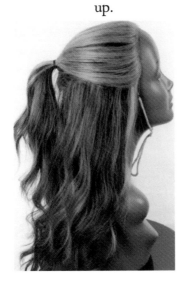

Step 3. After you have decided the placement of your up do, take a hair tie and make a ponytail. Twist your ponytail up into a bun and pin it securely using bobby pins.

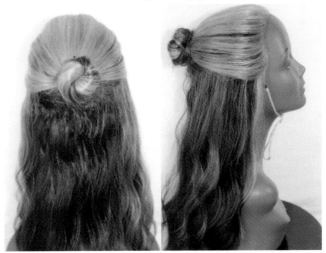

How to Create a Ponytail

<u>Tools Needed</u>
Wig Brush
Elastic Band
Holding Spray

Ponytails are simple to create. Pull all hair together, to the back center of head and secure it in place with a covered elastic band.

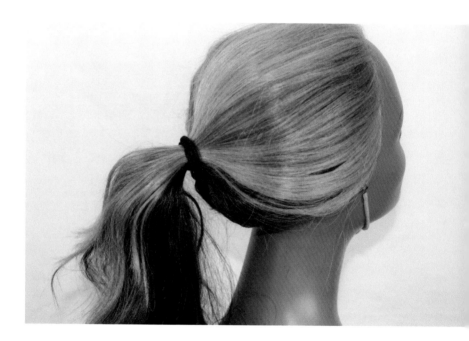

How to Create a Bouffant

Tools Needed

Hot Rollers

Comb

Wig Brush

Holding Spray

Step 1. Set the hair with large rollers.

Step 2. Remove the rollers, and tease the top of the hair.

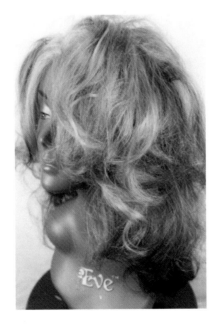

Step 3. After teasing the hair, smooth out the top layer of hair so the teased part is hidden and your hair looks rounded out. This style will also need to be held in place with holding spray.

After you have created your desired hairstyle, secure it with hair spray. The hair spray will prevent fly-away hair and will keep the hairstyle in place.

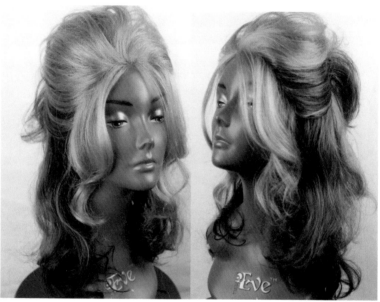

How to Keep Your Wig from Matting in the Back

Tools Needed

Silk or Satin Bonnet

Wide Tooth Comb

Wig Brush

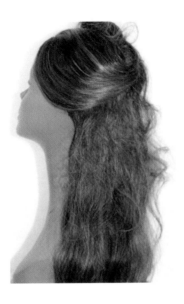

Wear a silk , satin bonnet or cap to bed. This will prevent matting of the hair while you sleep. Comb or brush the wig daily. Use a wide-tooth comb or wig brush to remove tangles and prevent matting.

Frequently Asked Questions

What should I use to brush or comb my wig? Use a brush that has single teeth from the base and has bristles that can flex or bend as they pass through the hair, this will lesson any possible damage

How can I detangle my wig? Leave In detangling conditioning spray is great on synthetic or human hair and is especially good for long hair and tight curled wigs.

What is the best way to wear my wig if I have long hair? There are three choices that work well for longer hair. Wrap the hair around the head and pin it in place underneath the wig. You can wear a wig cap. The wig cap fits tightly but comfortably over your hair and keeps your hair in place. You can also pin curl your hair under the wig.

Do I have to wear a wig cap? Using a wig cap is a personal preference. Most wig wearer's, whether they have long or short hair, prefer to use wig caps because it holds the hair in place better and helps to keep the wig cleaner.

What is the best choice for the hairline when the wig does not have bangs? Leave some of your hair out partially in the front then blend it into the wig so your own hairline is visible. This can be achieved when your own hair and the wig hair color blend together.

Can I go swimming with a lace wig on? Yes, use a strong bond if you choose to swim. Wash and condition your hair as soon as possible after swimming. Chlorine and saltwater can dry the hair out so using a good moisturizer is essential.

Can I wear my lace wig when I go to the gym and work out? Yes, you can wear your lace wig during any physical activity. It is a good idea to tie your hair down while you work out. Your adhesive may loosen a little as your body temperature rises however; it will set back in place as your body temperature cools down.

Will my hairline be damaged from adhesives? No follow the correct procedures used to remove your lace wig.

How can I prevent my lace wig from shedding? Knot sealer is the best way to prevent your wig from losing hair. Knot sealer is an acrylic based spray adhesive that coats the knots on your wig. We suggest spraying knot sealer on the inside of your lace wig each time after washing and allow your wig to air-dry on the wig head or stand.

Do I have to shave my hairline to wear a lace wig? No.

How do I choose the right adhesive and tape for my application? This depends on the length of time that you will like to wear your lace wig. Adhesives can have a hold time from 1-day to 6 weeks. You may have to try a few different adhesives before you find one that is perfect for your lifestyle. Everyone's body chemistry is different and what may work for one person may not necessarily work for the other.

How long can I keep my wig on? Lace wigs can be kept on until your adhesive loosens up. I don't recommend that you wear your lace wig beyond 2-3 weeks at a time because bacteria can build up from the adhesive and your natural production of oil.

How do I know what color is best suited for me? Use a color ring to select the color that matches you or the look you are trying to achieve.

How do I get my nape to stay secured? Many people have a problem with the nape area, because we are constantly moving our necks throughout the day. Securing the nape can easily be accomplished by adding bobby pins or wig combs to the area for a more secure fit.

How do I store my wig? The best way to store your wig is on a wig stand. This will help prevent your wig from becoming tangled or soiled between wearing. This also helps to maintain your wig's style and shape. Your wig should be stored in a clean, dry place, away from dust, mildew, and sources of high heat.

How do I know what style and length of wig is best for me? One of the best ways I recommend wig wearers to choose a wig style is to make a selection that best complements your facial shape. While some facial shapes look good with any wig, most must be carefully matched to a wig. Once you identify your face shape you'll be able to find the wig style that brings out the true beauty in your face.

Could a wig cause damage to my scalp, or slow my own natural hair growth? No, wearing a wig will not harm your scalp or inhibit new growth.

How often will I have to replace my wig? If you wear your wig every day it should be replaced every 3 months. If you wear your wig only once a week - then you will only need to replace it every 8 months.

Can I sleep in a wig? There are several options for sleeping in your wig. Use an older wig that has been worn during the day so that you preserve the life of your current wig worn during the day.

How do I care for my wig if I sleep in it at night? When caring for the wig that is worn at night each morning you brush all of the tangles from the hair. This will keep the hair from matting and frizzing up. The wig should be washed and conditioned at least once a week. Be sure to rinse the inside of the cap thoroughly to remove any excess shampoo or conditioner. Use a very thin cotton liner underneath the wig for comfort and to reduce the buildup of oils from the scalp on the inside of the cap. Other alternatives that are options are a synthetic wig that has a cotton head band attached, a less expensive synthetic wig, or a less expensive human hair wig that is light weight. Also a lighter density of hair will be cooler and more comfortable for sleeping.

Can I use a blow dryer on my synthetic wig? No. Excessive heat will melt or frizz the plastic in your wig's fibers.

Wig Terms & Glossary

Accent Color - A sharp, intense color used as a contrast or pickup for color scheme to add excitement to the hair.

Adjustable Tabs – Tabs that allow you to adjust your wig with hooks or velcro at the nape section for a better fit.

Baby Hairs – Fine, short or curled hairs, ventilated in the opposite direction of the wig placed around the perimeter of a wig to give the wig a more natural look.

Backcombing- A term for teasing hair, the hair is combed down towards the scalp in order to create more volume or a rooted hair line creating a matting effect and forming a cushion at the base of the hair.

Bangs - Hair that is cut to fall over the forehead.

Bleach -A method used to lighten hair color.

Body – The volume or springiness of hair.

Bonding – To attach wefted hair to the wig with glue or other adhesives.

Bob - Cutting all of the hair chin length.

Bobby pin - Thin metal or plastic expandable, ridged clips used to hold and secure the hair into a style

Bouffant – Big voluminous hair.

Blocking a Wig - The act of securing a wig to a block so that the wig is secure and ready to be worked on.

Blow Dryer- Hand held tool for drying and styling hair.

Blunt Cut- Cutting the hair to one equal length.

Braid - To interlace strands of hair to form a pattern.

Bulk Hair -A bundle of loose hair with no weft or track.

Cap – The foundation or base of a wig which the hair is attached.

Chin Straps – Jaws clips that go underneath your chin and attaches to your wig cap on both sides and makes styling wigs easier.

Cleaning the Wig - The act of cleaning the glue, residue and makeup off the wig.

Clips- Small hinged hair clips that are used as a styling aid.

Classic Style – A hair design that has enduring popularity.

Corn Rows- A row of braids that are divided into sections and are braided together tightly close to the scalp.

Coarse Hair – A description for stronger, thicker types of hair.

Conditioner – Creamy hair product used after shampooing that helps to moisturize and detangle hair.

Couture Cut – A high fashion hair cut that is exclusively tailored to your lifestyle or wardrobe.

Crown - The top part of the head.

Curl – The portion of the strand that is wound into a falling circle by heat or processing.

Curling Iron- Cylindrical electric devise, of various diameters, used to curl the hair.

Custom Wig – A wig made with any combination of hair fiber, cap, style or color to get you exactly what you want in a wig that is designed specifically for you.

Deep Penetrating Treatment – A conditioner for occasional use that contains protein, vitamins and moisture to help dry, damaged hair.

Density – The number of hair per square inch on the scalp.

Duck Bill Clips- A type of a clip used in styling, that is about 3 inches long and opens like a ducks bill to clamp onto the hair.

Elasticity – The hairs ability to stretch without breaking and return to its natural state.

Feathering – Cutting technique used to take the hard lines out of the hair by cutting softer lines.

Finish – The final step in a hairstyle, final placement of strands and application of the hair.

Foundation- The base shape of a head that aids in creating custom wigs.

Flat Iron- A heating iron that has two flat plates that the hair is pulled through in order to straighten it.

Freezing Spray – Hair spray with the firmest hold used to maintain the style of hard to hold hair.

Gel – Jelly like material formed by the coagulation of a liquid, used to aid the hair in holding its shape.

Growth Pattern- The direction that a person's hair grows, it is unique to each person.

German Lace- A stronger lace with hexagonal holes

Hand Tied/ Hand Made Wigs – A wig or hairpiece which the hair has been knotted into the base of the cap. Handmade tops may have a machine made cap and the top is hand tied to allow more versatility.

Hair Cutting Shears- Scissor that are specifically made for cutting hair.

Hair Extensions- Hair that is attached using glue, hair braiding, or sewing the hair into the head or wig.

Hair Fibers – A mixture of human hair, synthetic hair or some combination of hair that is knotted, glued or sewn into a wig cap.

Hair Line- The line around the face where the hair begins to grow.

Hair Piece- Any piece of artificial hair that does not cover the entire head.

Highlights – The subtle lifting of color in specific sections of hair.

Humidity – The amount of moisture available in the air.

Holding Spray – Hair spray with medium hold used to make hair maintain its shape.

Invisible Thread - A clear nylon thread, used for sewing together hair to a wig cap.

Kosher Wigs – Contain no hair from India.

Lace Front Wig – A wig with the front made of lace material for versatility and off the face parting.

Layering – Is a technique used to change the thickness of the hair, creating either a thinning or thicker appearance.

Long Wigs – Wigs that go past the shoulder.

Machine Made Wig Caps – Wefted wigs made by machine.

Medium Wigs – Wigs that are below the ear but above the shoulders.

Monofilament Material- A lacey material that is used in monofilament wig caps

Nape - The back of the neck, at the base of the hairline.

Non Remy Hair- Hair that has been stripped of its cuticle and is coated with silicone and other chemicals to mimic the softness and shine of virgin Remy hair.

Petite Wigs – Wigs for a person with a head size of 20 ½ to 21 ½, it does mean short wig.

Permanent Hair Color – Completely changing the natural color of the hair.

Pin Curl – A type of curl where the hair is rolled flat into a circle and secured with bobby pins or clips. Pin curls are used as both a styling technique and a way to prep the hair for a wig to be place over it.

Plait- One complete step in the braiding sequence.

Pre Styled Wig – A wig that has a basic cut and curl pattern already in it, and requires minimum work.

Processed Hair – Human Hair that has been chemically treated or colored.

Reconditioning A Wig – To clean and add de frizz conditioner, and bring a wig back to life using a professional cleaning method.

Resistant – Hair that repels liquids and chemicals lacks manageability.

Restyling – Taking a pre-styled wig and changing its appearance by cutting, adding hair or changing the way it falls.

Roots – The part of the hair that is attached to the scalp.

Sectioning- Dividing the portion of hair you plan to work with from the rest of the hair.

Shag – A hair cut that is choppy and layered all over.

Short Wigs – Wigs that are above the ears.

Steaming A Wig – The act of applying steam to a synthetic wig in order to either straighten the hair fibers or set the curl into the hair fibers

Strands - Sections of hair that are twisted together to form a braid.

Styled Wig – A wig that has had extended work done on it by a stylist. Most wigs especially human hair need additional work done on them.

Tendril – A small, thin curling wisp of hair often located around the face.

Thinning Shears – A special type of hair cutting scissors in which one of the blades is notched so that all the hair is not cut.

Tips – The part of the hair shaft that is farthest away from the scalp. The ends of the hair on the wig.

Ultra Hold- Lace wig adhesive

Ultra Petite Wig – A wig for a person with a head size of 19 ½ to 20 ½ inches.

Under looping or Under venting – Adding strands of hair just under the front edge of a wig to hide the cap.

Unstyled Wig – A wig in its natural state that requires cutting, styling to look as one wants.

Up do- A hairstyle that's pinned and arranged up and off the shoulders and neck.

Virgin Hair – Refers to human hair that is still in its original state from the donors head

Venting- The space between the wefts on a wig for ventilation to keep the head cooler and make the wig more comfortable.

Ventilating – The act of knotting hair to a wig lace to give the appearance that the hair is growing directly from the scalp.

Ventilating Needle – A hook that is shaped like a crochet needle and is used to grab the hair to be knotted onto a wig.

Volume – The degree to which the hair extends from the head in a finished hair style.

Weft – An amount of hair or fiber that is doubled over and MACHINE-SEWN along the top to create a long strand of hair, held together by a "track" or "weft" that has been stitched to the hair.

Wig Block- A block made of wood or other material shaped like a head that is used to mount wigs for construction or styling.

Wig Clips – Clips that are sewn into a wig, or hair piece that snaps and lock to the hair to ensure a secure attachment.

Wig Clamp - A device that clamps to a table edge and has a post that a wig block sits on.

Wig Dryer- Large wooden boxes with a current of warm air flowing through them used to dry wigs.

Wig Let- A hairpiece that consists of a small circle of hair mounted on a round base used to fill in thin places of the hair or to add a little volume to a hairstyle.

Wig Prep- The act of preparing a person's hair as flat as possible to their head so that the wig can be placed over it.

Wig Stand – A metal stand about 3 feet high with adjustable height that the wig block or head attaches to for leveled wig making and styling.

Wig Making Order Form

Sample

Type of Wig Cap:

Nylon Cap	Standard Cap	¾ Cap	Dome Cap	Lace Front Cap	Mono-filament Cap

Type of Hair:

Human Hair	Synthetic Hair	Hair Blend

Color of Hair:

2 Black	4 Brown	6 Light Brown	27 Blonde	613 Platinum Blonde

Details of Wig:

Length:

Density:

Front: Temple: Crown: Nape:

Hair Cut:

Length of Part:

Left: Center: Right:

Part Location:

Left: Center: Right:

Notes or Specific Instructions:

Where to Order Wig Making Tools

Available at Wal-Mart
Blow Dryer
Hand sewing needles
Holding Spray
Different colors of thread
Soft tape measure
Spritz
Something to put your ventilating needles in
Seam ripper
Small sharp scissors
Small needle nose pliers
Curling iron
Flat iron
Gel
Spritz
Pin Cushion
Hand Held Steamer
Mist Bottle

Available at HisandHer.com
Human Hair
Synthetic Hair
Wig Caps (Standard, Monofilament, Lace Front Wig Caps)
Ventilating needles
Needle Holder
Wig T-pins
Wig Blocks

Available at Your Local Beauty Supply Store

Wire mesh rollers

Bobby Pins

Hair Pins

Hot Rollers

Duckbill clips

Wig Clips

Wig Combs

Teasing Brush

Wig Brush with wire bristles

Rattail Comb

Small tooth comb

30 Second Bonding Glue and Remover

007 Bonding Weave Crème

Ultra Hold wig adhesive and remover

Liquid Gold wig adhesive and remover

Available at Wimexbeauty.com

Wig Stand Tripod

Table top wig holder

Mannequin Heads

Wig Heads

LookofLove.com

Chin Straps

Notes

CPSIA information can be obtained
at www.ICGtesting.com
Printed in the USA
LVIC04n1357160614
390252LV00002B/6